It's no... ...that
kills us, it's our
reaction to it

- Hans Selye
the father of stress

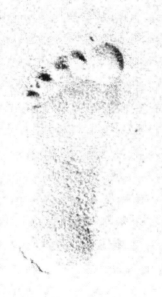

Models used in this book are the author's own, namely:

- SPEAR model: Summarising the Stress Response
- Your Stress Support Structure - Making Rooms in your Life
- Climbing Everest illustration

(I'm quite proud of these, feel free to talk about them as interesting models that have helped you understand and relate to your own stress situation.)

Royalty-free images from Pixabay and Unsplash.

This book comes with a relaxation audio to help reduce stress - if you want a copy of the download, send an email to geraldine@mind-yourbusiness.co.uk and you'll be sent a link with information on how to use it. It will help you sleep better which helps you manage stress and your capacity to cope with more 'stuff'.

CONTENTS

INTRODUCTION

What's in this book..?

Understanding your personal stress footprint is a bit like knowing what kind of foods you love and hate, it's integral to your character, your spirit, the very 'you-ness' of you. And yet few people spend time getting to know themselves, knowing what their stress triggers are, what their strategies could be to prevent them being overwhelmed and understanding how it all fits together life a jigsaw...

But that's about to change for you - because this short e-book will lift the lid on the stress response system which will enable you to move from emotional reactions that you seem not to have any control over, to being more considered and proactive.

Imagine being able to choose your emotional reactions so that you become the calm Zen master of all decision-making, admired for your cool-headedness and ability to see beyond the immediate situation?

What if you rarely lose your cool in front of your children?

How would you feel if your friends and family look to you with admiration at your abilities to juggle work, home, life so effortlessly?

It's all possible through re-training your brain, building resilience to stress and living your best life.

Stop waiting for the children to grow up, the project to finish, retirement to come... get off that 'head-down, keep going' treadmill, and start making positive decisions that work for you.

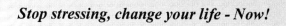

Stop stressing, change your life - Now!

How to use this book

This is not a big book, in fact you could read it in less than an hour but it has exercises that need some thought. I wanted to keep it short and quick to read, so you actually benefit from every page. Through the mix of information and exercises you really can change your life - I know because I use them in real life situations with my clients, both as a clinical hypnotherapist specialising in stress management and as a stress consultant working with organisations what want to make their workplaces well.

Skim through it first, then go back and do the exercises, refer back to pages (there are notes about referring back in certain places), and follow the 7 days to start climbing your mountain plan. We're all a work in progress so you might as well make sure your foundations are solid for the next several decades!

In order to truly understand the real causes of **stress**, we need to understand how we function. By understanding how we work as humans, we can then look at practical strategies to promote good mental health - to live your best life.

In this book we will be unpacking what stress and mental health means, look into how the brain works and the effects on our physiology, as well as the anatomy of stress - what happens when we're under too much pressure, the cracks that may appear.

Through a series of exercises you can work out what your personal stress triggers are, what you can do to alleviate them and how to build your tolerance - because there is no such thing as being stress-free.

Life happens, the important thing is to be able to cope when stress builds up and enjoy thriving the rest of the time!

"You can't stop the waves, but you can learn to surf"

- Jon Kabat-Zinn

ABOUT THE AUTHOR:
Geraldine Joaquim DipM DSFH HPD

Having spent over 20 years working in international marketing, Geraldine Joaquim made a complete change in career direction, she went off the deep end, got in touch with her previously-unknown spiritual side and retrained as a hypnotherapist. She continued slogging away in corporate alongside building her private practice before she stopped messing around and went into stress management full time.

She brings together her skills as a presenter, bowling people over with her wit and insights, with her learnings focused on the neuroscience of the stress response system, plus her personal experiences in a stressful work environment, running the gamut from bullying managers to fights in airline queues, not to mention the passive-aggressive actions of various hotel housekeeping staff in not leaving her room as she liked it...

Geraldine is keen to promote stress prevention as the key to good health (with a healthy dose of humour): it's not about avoiding pressure but how we cope that makes the difference, and she has an innate belief that everyone deserves to be happy at work which also benefits the companies they work for. Her motto is 'when you can get the donkey to want to do the work, you don't need the carrot or the stick!' (or something along those lines because describing employees as donkeys isn't very nice).

But beyond simply coping with stress and building resilience, lies thriving – that state of being that we can all attain, when we are living our best lives not role-playing zombies in the Land of the Living Dead.
She has gone on to deliver workshops and talks in diverse organisations including ParkNow, a technology division of BMW, University of Surrey,

Office of the Police & Crime Commissioner for Surrey, Institute of Directors, as well as sitting on expert panels such as the Un-learn event sponsored by Adaptai. She has featured as an expert voice in the media including Men's Health, BBC News, Metro (under her own author by-line no less), HRNews and Glassdoor, she has been involved in 'How to Break into the Elite' a BBC2 programme due to air in July 2019, and 'The Why Factor' from BBC World Service radio, and provides content for wellness and leadership platforms such as QDOOS.

As well as seeing people privately for stress management, writing content, giving talks and workshops, Geraldine fits in being married, two children, a dog, a cat, two rabbits and two guinea pigs at the moment, the number of animals fluctuates from time to time. She often confuses all their names. She runs to keep her head clear, has completed the London Marathon (she didn't win but the flapjacks she took with her helped), competed in a few 10kms races and in a few triathlons.

She puts out quite a lot of content on Linked In and always welcomes new contacts so feel free to send her a connection request (you don't have to send a message but it would be nice, especially if you want to tell her how much you enjoyed this book)...

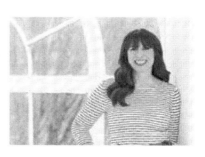

https://www.linkedin.com/in/geraldinejoaquim/

CHAPTER 1:
BACKGROUND TO STRESS

*"If you can keep your head when all about you
Are losing theirs and blaming it on you,
If you can trust yourself when all men doubt you,
But make allowance for their doubting too."*

- Rudyard Kipling

If you're suffering from stress, you're not alone...

In the UK we are suffering from an epidemic of stress:

- 595,000 workers suffering from work-related stress, depression or anxiety (new or long-standing) in 2017/18, an increase of over 13% on 2016/17 at 526,000 workers [note 1/1A]

- 57% of days lost to ill-health attributed to stress, depression or anxiety in 2017/18, an increase of 16% on 2016/17 at 49% of days lost [note 1/1A]

- 15.4mn working days lost due to work-related stress, depression or anxiety in 2017/18, an increase of 23% on 2016/17 at 12.5mn working days lost [note 1/1A]

- £70-£100bn estimated cost of mental health problems to UK economy (account for 4.5% of GDP) [note 2]

- 300,000 workers lose their jobs annually due to mental health issues [note 3]

- Poor mental health costs UK employers up to £42bn [note 3]

Notes
(1) HSE http://www.hse.gov.uk/statistics/causdis/stress/ 2016/17
(1A) HSE http://www.hse.gov.uk/statistics/overall/hssh1718.pdf 2017/18
(2) Department of Health: Annual Report of the Chief Medical Officer 2013
https://www.gov.uk/government/publications/chief-medical-officer-cmo-annual-report-public-mental-health
(3) Stevenson Farmer 'Thriving at Work' report, Oct 2017
https://assets.publishing.service.gov.uk/government/uploads/system/uploads/attachment_data/file/658145/thriving-at-work-stevenson-farmer-review.pdf
(4) NHS Information Centre for health and social care
http://webarchive.nationalarchives.gov.uk/20180328130852tf_/http://content.digital.nhs.uk/data-and-information/publications/statistical/adult-psychiatric-morbidity-survey/adult-psychiatric-morbidity-in-england-2007-results-of-a-household-survey/

The individual context...

- Approximately 1 in 4 people in the UK will experience a mental health problem each year (note 4)
- In England, 1 in 6 people report experiencing a common mental health problem (such as anxiety and depression) in any given week (note 5)
- 53% of all employees feel uncomfortable talking about mental health issues like depression and anxiety at work at all (note 6)
- 13% of employees feel they can't disclose a mental health issue to their line manager (note 6)

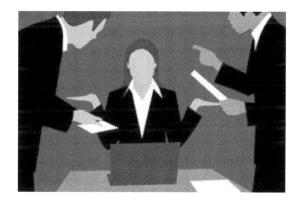

Notes
 (5) NHS
http://webarchive.nationalarchives.gov.uk/20180328140249/http://digital.nhs.uk/catalogue/PUB21748
(6) Deloitte Monitor https://www2.deloitte.com/content/dam/Deloitte/uk/Documents/public-sector/deloitte-uk-mental-health-employers-monitor-deloitte-oct-2017.pdf

What's happening in the background?

Newspapers, social media, radio, TV, internet, apps... all these things form part of the background to our lives. We might not recognise any the headlines per se but as a whole they will be familiar.

- Feb 2018: Antidepressants work! A study which analysed data found 21 common anti-depressants were all more effective at reducing symptoms of acute depression than placebos – however whether we need them to be prescribed on a mass basis is another story.
- Daily Mail (Dec 29 2017): the UK is now ranked 4th out of 29 western nations for prescribing antidepressants
- 2016 record 64.7mn antidepressants prescribed (that's 108.5% increase in the last decade)

GP's are trying to deal with a mental health tidal wave offering 'quick fixes'. It is estimated that stress-related conditions now make up the majority of GP caseloads – it's not because they don't care about their patients, they simply don't have the resources in either time or money to find out what the real causes are behind the symptoms presented.

Things are changing...

The 2017 London Marathon was the springboard for the Royal Foundation's Head's Together campaign, aired on BBC's 'Mind over Marathon' programme – this also prompted the government to make a public commitment to dealing with mental health.

Back in January 2017, the government commissioned an independent review into mental health in the workplace, which was published in October 2017, the **Thriving at Work Report** which released 6 key points:

1. Produce, implement and communicate a mental health at work plan

2. Develop mental health awareness among employees

3. Encourage open conversations about mental health and the support available when employees are struggling

4. Provide your employees with good working conditions

5. Promote effective people management

6. Routinely monitor employee mental health and wellbeing

CHAPTER 2:
BUT WHAT IS STRESS?

It all started with Hans Selye, a pioneering endocrinologist who explained his stress model based on physiology and psychobiology as the General Adaptation Syndrome (GAS), a response of the body to demands placed upon it. As a medical student, he noticed that patients suffering from different diseases often exhibited identical signs and symptoms. This observation may have been the first step in his recognition of "stress". His work details how stress causes hormonal responses which can, over time, lead to long term conditions such as ulcers, high blood pressure, arthritis, allergic reactions and kidney disease. His landmark article was published in 1936.

You might be surprised to learn that the term 'stress' was first coined by Selye only a little more than 50 years ago, yet it has become an ingrained part of our vocabulary and daily existence.

"Without stress, there would be no life"
- Hans Seyle

Humans in particular thrive on stress, it is key to our survival. We need it to get up in the morning, it motivates us to achieve bigger and better things, to win new clients, it pushes us forward. But too much stress can be detrimental, weakening the immune system causing symptoms like high blood pressure, fatigue, anxiety and depression, it can cause internal inflammation leading to heart disease, diabetes, not to mention any number of other physical and mental signs developing.

So what causes 'bad' stress?

In our modern world we tend to operate on Auto-pilot - we get caught in a **'Driven-Doing' mode** that is:

- Habitually responsive/reactive
- Over-analysing
- Continually striving
- Seeing thoughts and feelings as solid and 'real'
- Aversion to difficulty
- Mental time travel (past/future, not the now)

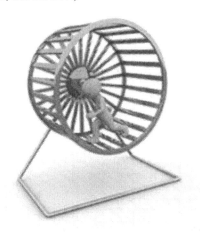

In this Driven-Doing Mode you might find yourself...

- Running on automatic without much awareness of what you're doing (in routines, doing what we've always done, head down and get on)

- Rushing through activities without being really attentive to them (eating, being with loved ones)

- Having a tendency not to notice physical tension or discomfort until it really grabs your attention (tension in shoulders, painful joints, avoiding getting things checked out)

- Preoccupied with the future or the past (dwelling on past actions, thinking ahead to the next job)

- Listening to someone with one ear, whilst thinking about something else at the same time (very common when dealing with children - and partners!)

From the Mindful Attention and Awareness Scale
- Brown & Ryan, 2003

Additionally, our environment has changed considerably: our consumption of information has increased 350% in 30 years and we are in an age of 'continuous partial attention' exacerbated by technology.

And we have a common misconception that we can multi-task – in fact we have become adept at switching our attention between tasks but it's exhausting for our brains, and is in itself stressful!

Does any of this sound familiar?

CHAPTER 3:
OUR BRILLIANT BUT IMPERFECT BRAINS

Evolution vs. Revolution

In order to understand stress we need to consider the circumstances behind it's development as a system, it's importance to our survival as a species.

Humans have been in development for around 5-6,000,000 years, way back to our most primitive primate ancestors

Our current form (homo sapiens) evolved 100-150,000 years ago

Civilisation is roughly 6,000 years old - the Sumerians of Mesopotamia, thought to have formed the first human civilisation, lived in southern Mesopotamia between the Tigris and Euphrates Rivers in the Middle East. They built villages and cities, cultivated crops and practised animal husbandry, shared common language and developed Cuneiform writing initially to record business transactions and keep tallies but eventually it became a fully-fledged writing system, used for everything from poetry and literature to history and law. They used a number system based on 60 which is still used today: the origins of the 60 second minute and 60 minute hour can be traced back to ancient Mesopotamia

Our modern working life was devised around 200 years ago, during the Industrial Revolution: 8 hours for work, 8 hours for recreation, 8 hours for rest. The 40-hour week was a social movement to regulate the length of a working day, preventing excesses and abuses at a time when 10-12 hour working days were not uncommon but were unsustainable, especially given the lack of proper nutrition and poor housing many labours suffered.

The Digital Revolution, between 1950 and the late 1970's, saw the shift from mechanical and analogue technology to digital electronics, and the adoption of digital computers and digital record keeping

Our current Technological Age which started just 20-30 years ago has seen sweeping changes in the way we live our lives - the rise of technology in the form of mobile phones, personal computers and laptops, tablets, the way information and knowledge is accessed, all have seen huge changes in the way we connect with others and live our lives. And it's an era of misinformation,

Evolution takes time but the pace of change in our modern environment has happened in the blink of an eye! Compare the 5-6 million years of evolution we have gone through to get to our current form with just (at best) 6,000 years of civilisation, not to mention the huge changes we have seen in recent years - our brains haven't noticed the wallpaper has changed.

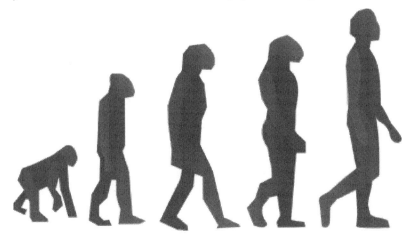

Your brain is hardwired for survival not happiness.

The human brain has developed with the sole purpose of getting us through today so we live again tomorrow, it's not interested in your happiness or self-esteem or self-actualisation - it's all about survival!

Primitive Brain in a modern world

Our primitive ancestors lived in a world full of danger - whether it was a predator, a marauding tribe or the elements, every time they popped their heads outside their cave they faced life-or-death situations.

The worse situations we face now come from bad traffic, running late, trains being delayed, the bank statement arriving, arguments at work or home, deadlines, dealing with tricky clients or truculent children, spilling our coffee... they represent barriers to us getting our needs met throughout the day, they are cumulative and they are taken on board by the primitive part of our brain as threats to life. They activate the same stress response system as if they are life-or-death situations - which isn't very helpful.

Let's take a look at your brain...

If you think of your brain being split roughly into 2 halves: the top part is your rational, logical, intellectual brain, the part you use for learning, planning, interacting with the world, it's where you make rational, positive decisions based on a proper assessment of the situation.

Then there's the other part, the emotional primitive part, which is solely concerned with your survival.

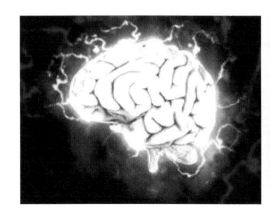

It looks after your autonomic functions like your heart rate, breathing, oxygen exchange, temperature control - all the things that need to happen to keep you alive that you don't actually think about (because if you h ad to think about them, you probably wouldn't last very long) - and it looks after your security, keeping you safe from all those things that could be out to get you.

This is where you will find your freeze-flight-fight response centre, the amygdala, and it works together with the hippocampus (basically a pattern matching system containing all of your learned - and sometimes inappropriate - behaviours and experiences), and the hypothalamus which regulates the chemical response in your body and mind.

The amygdala is constantly scanning the environment for any threats to life, it never switches off that's why if you hear a bump in the night you're immediately awake (some people have different sensitivities to others).

In the primitive days of our ancestors, if they came across a predatory animal this part of the brain would immediately leap to action, the amygdala would refer to the hippocampus for a pattern match (in this case, there would be one and it is fierce!), and it would simultaneously activate the hypothalamus to release cortisol, the stress hormone, and adrenaline to prepare the body for action.

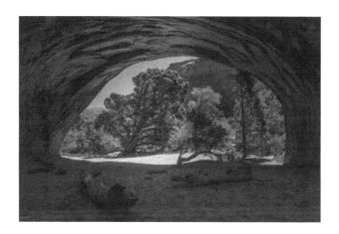

Your ancestor would notice their palms go sweaty, their heart rate increase and their stomach might be churning, they might even evacuate their bowels, a natural part of the stress response as it gets rid of extraneous 'baggage', gets them ready to act – all physical symptoms of what we might recognise today as stress.

So, the survival mode is vital and works well for specific incidents that we can respond to but under prolonged stress, so-called non-essential processes like digestion and reproduction are turned off, as the body is focused on being ready to shut down, run or fight

It's a necessarily simple system that is highly effective, and it's the reason you are sitting here reading this today! Your ancestors used this system to stay alive - well, at least long enough to procreate.

We can map the process out as follows:

Your amygdala is constantly scanning the environment for threats to life (translated from anything that acts as a barrier to you getting what you want, or pushing you out of your comfort zone, or change), it detects a STIMULUS.

It refers to the hippocampus, your onboard filing cabinet which stores all your templates of behaviour, for a PATTERN MATCH. If there's a match with positive behaviour attached, the amygdala moves back to scanning mode, if there's a negative match or no template, it triggers EMOTIONAL arousal, causing the hypothalamus to release cortisol, the stress hormone, to get you ready for ACTION (freeze-flight-fight).

And once the situation passes, the behaviour or actions you have just displayed will REINFORCE the template, marking it as appropriate for future reference.

It can be described as the SPEAR model.

SPEAR model – understanding the process of stress

THE SPEAR MODEL

S — STIMULUS
The primitive brain constantly scans the environment for perceived threat. Stimulus detected

P — PATTERN MATCHING
Subconscious referral to the hippocampus for a pattern match or template of behaviour to form a response to the stimulus, based on our previous experiences and learned behaviours

E — EMOTIONAL AROUSAL
Triggered by pattern match:
- Positive template match causes the system to loop back to start
- Negative or no template causes stress hormones to be released

A — ACTION
In the case of perceived threat the brain always falls back on the Freeze - Flight - Fight response (which we can translate into modern-day symptoms of depression / anxiety / anger)

R — REINFORCE TEMPLATE
Successful action that preserves life reinforces that template as 'appropriate' for future reference

Your Primitive Opt-out Clauses of Freeze - Flight - Fight

If the primitive brain thinks your life is in some sort of emergency or crisis, it will step in to help - which is useful if we're facing life-or-death situations but not so good when it's a traffic light turning red, or a looming deadline or a relationship breakdown.

The cumulative effect of these trickling irritants builds and the stress response system steps in more frequently, it ratchets up the stress levels and releases more and more cortisol and adrenaline into your system, which becomes hyper-sensitive - now, it's almost as if you're looking for stress, looking for a fight.

Your system always relies on the primitive opt-out clauses of freeze - flight - fight, either solely or using a combination of all three.

Freeze - depression

Imagine being your primitive ancestor, looking out on a world full of danger, perhaps there's a predator outside or the weather is bad. You can't go out to hunt so the best thing you can do is to hunker down, withdraw into yourself to conserve your energy and ride out the time until the situation changes - and we've translated this into the modern-day symptoms of **depression**. Unfortunately our modern world does not readily allow for hunkering down, for duvet days, so we battle through low periods but don't really address them

Flight - anxiety

If you were living in the wilds, you would probably be on red alert at all times, living on your wits and being **anxious** about every shadow, every noise around you, being ready to flee.

Fight - anger

And **anger** is merely a primitive way of increasing our strength, making us bigger and stronger so that we can defend ourselves against other tribes or wild animals.

But there's more: the primitive brain has a **negative default**. If you did face a wild animal you wouldn't want to spent any time debating whether it looks hungry, whether it might be interested in eating you - no, you would want to take immediate action so it is necessarily negatively biased to preserve your life ("It's going to eat you, get out of there!")

It's also **obsessional** - if you faced dangers every day you would be wise to check and re-check your environment constantly. So if you find yourself double-checking the front door is locked, don't worry, it's perfectly normal. It's just that primitive urge to make sure everything is as it should be, to check your safety. It only becomes a problem if it takes you 3 hours to leave the house each day because you're checking and re-checking everything several times!

And it's **vigilant**. If there's a perception of danger around you, you'd be wise to stay on red alert - if you feel stress in one part of your life, invariably you'll be stressed in other areas because that primitive brain is looking for trouble...

This part of the brain is not an intellect.

The primitive brain cannot come up with new ideas all by itself, it relies on past patterns of behaviour. If what got you through today worked and you survived, then you'll be encouraged to do it again, and that's how habits are formed whether they're good ones or bad ones.

Say you've had a stressful day at work. You get home and head straight to the fridge, you get out a bottle of wine and pore yourself a glass. It goes down nicely, you can feel yourself unwind, the stress eases and you feel ready to get on with your evening.

The next time you feel stressed at work, your primitive brain pushes forward that action (drinking a glass of wine) as a great antidote to the stress so as soon as you get home you head to the fridge, you're not even thinking consciously about it, you just do it - and it works again.

This is how habits are formed - action without thought - and sometimes we create habits that are not helpful, that are not consciously developed, they just happen. Before you know it, you're having that glass of wine more frequently and the problem is, one glass doesn't keep hitting the spot because your system quickly becomes accustomed to the effects of that one glass of alcohol, it starts to need more to feel the same effects so one glass becomes two, then three, then it's a whole bottle and a regular trip to the bottle bank...

At no point did your primitive brain understand that the mere act of getting home and doing a simple action, any action at all that moves your thoughts from stressful work to more pleasant ones associated with being at home, is the real point of reducing stress. The fact that this particular one involved alcohol is irrelevant, but it becomes the hook that you find yourself caught on.

Life happens all around us, it's a series of ups and downs with a little bit of freewheeling in the middle! People cope with stress in different ways and, as mentioned before, humans can actually thrive on stress.

We can translate it into the state of our mental health – stress and mental health are inextricably linked. Positive mental health is rarely an absolute state, it is highly unlikely that anyone feels happy all the time: factors both in and out of work affect the mental health of everyone, moving us up or down a spectrum that ranges from good to poor – just like our physical health changes from feeling 100% fit to catching a cold or having aches and pains.

You might generally have positive mental health but a problem at home may trigger a period of low mood or even depression moving you into poor mental health. Or you may be living with a mental health condition, such as depression or phobias, but with coping strategies that are working well and mean you move into having positive mental health.

Throughout our lives, we move through a continual wave of feeling ok, moving up into anxiety and down into depression.

This is normal.

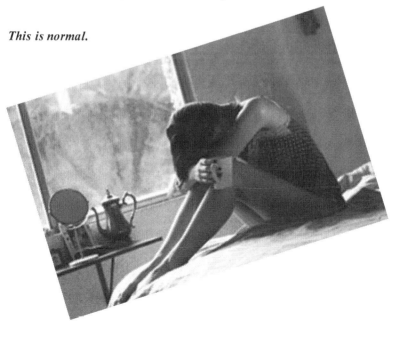

However, we sometime go through periods of stress that result in longer term low mood, feelings of anger or anxiety – but one thing is a constant: life happens! So it is not practical to avoid stress altogether, it's about building **resilience to cope** that is important.

And it's important to understand that it is often not the actual situations we face that causes much of our stress but how we think about it, it's the thought patterns we have rather than reality.

I'd like you to consider a roomful of students sitting their exams - the majority of them will feel a little nervous but they'll get their heads down and get on with the paper in front of them.

A small percentage will feel more anxious, they'll struggle to focus but they will get through.

But a handful of students will really struggle, they might feel physically sick, feel faint, their hands will shake, they're on the verge of panic, they can't read the paper properly. The whole situation is a real nightmare for them, they just can't perform well.

Now, every student in this scene is facing the same thing yet it is down to their individual thought patterns that dictates whether they sail through the exams or if they sink into a black hole of nerves. So it is not necessarily the events in our lives that causes the perception of crisis - it's our thought patterns surrounding those events, and every negative thought we have is converted into anxiety.

We create anxiety by negatively forecasting the big stuff in life (remember the primitive brain's propensity for negativity), things like getting promotions, landing clients, personal relationships, health, etc, and the small things: will the traffic be okay on my way to work, will that meeting go well, will the client like my work?

You might think about these things over and over again, endlessly ruminating on the negative outcomes.

All these thoughts activate exactly the same system as if they're real, so the stress response system goes on standby, it ratchets up the anxiety levels, releases cortisol and adrenaline, gets you ready for action (freeze, flight, fight). In the end the actual event is fine, the traffic is good, the client loves your work, the meeting goes well... but you've 'been through it' numerous times in your mind with negative outcomes in comparison to the one actual good result.

And unless you've lived a life of total peace and solitude, there will be stuff in the past that you ruminate on, all those 'would haves, could haves, if only's we negatively introspect about.

Remember when we're in an auto-pilot mode we have a tendency to 'time travel', spending a lot of our time thinking about the past and future but not being present in the 'now'.

Real or imagined, it all goes into our **STRESS BUCKET**...

The Stress Bucket

Imagine you have a metaphorical bucket sitting in your head and all those negative thoughts, whether about real events or imagined ones, go into it throughout the day. Over time it fills up.

As the bucket gets fuller you might notice some physical or emotional symptoms building up, perhaps tension in your muscles or headaches, maybe feeling tearful or angry, perhaps skin rashes or an upset stomach.

Eventually, if you don't do anything about it, your bucket will overflow - and that's when you go into meltdown whether it's having a panic attack, freezing on the spot or even a full-on psychotic episode (psychosis is a mental health problem that causes people to perceive or interpret things differently from those around them, they have an altered version of reality, and it might involve hallucinations or delusions).

Most of us bubble along with partially full buckets, sometimes having small episodes of emotional outbursts or having physical health problems because stress affects our immune systems. The level rises and falls depending on the pressure we're under.

When we have rather too much in our bucket, we might over-react to small problems - say you've had a bad day at work, you're bucket is fuller than normal and when you get home your son or daughter spills a cup of water - you find yourself getting really cross, shouting, out of proportion to the actual spill. It's an indication that your bucket is full - it's not about the spilled water, it about the stuff that's happened before that point.

Resilience is simply having space in your bucket.

The more 'space' you have in your bucket, the more capacity you have to take on more, to cope better.

There are 2 ways of dealing with your stress bucket:

1) Stop filling it

Every time you find yourself thinking about something going wrong in the future or a negative outcome, stop and bring your attention back to the present. Remember that all those negative thoughts don't do anything, they don't change anything, they just fill your bucket which is both useless and harmful to you.

2) Empty it

Thankfully we have an effective way of emptying our stress bucket - during the REM (Rapid Eye Movement) phase of sleep. At night we re-run the events of the day/week/month/year and change them from being an emotional memory to a narrative one - a memory that we have control over.

It works like this: imagine you've had an argument at work, you're really upset and you're still thinking about it when you go to bed that night. During the REM phase of sleep your brain will re-run the event either in clear (as it actually happened) or metaphorically , a story that your brain creates around the event which may also pull in other experiences from the past, people or scenes from TV or a movie, mashing it all together into a surreal dream that seems completely disjointed or bizarre - effectively your brain is playing with the memory, deciding if it needs to keep it in your bucket or whether it can move it to your long term memory banks, removing the emotional aspect of it.

It might take a few nights to work through, depending on the impact of the argument, but by the end of the week if a colleague asks you about it, you can relay the event without feeling upset - you still remember it but it is no longer in the forefront of your mind and no longer has the emotional attachment. This is the same system that helps us through bereavement, we don't forget our loved ones but we can begin to remember and talk about them without the emotional arousal their loss engenders. It's a very necessary process that enables us to carry on without huge emotional burdens that would cripple us and jeopardise our survival.

Unfortunately REM is restricted to around 20% of our sleep pattern. During times of high stress you might have too much to process through and once the quota is up, your mind wakes you up - you find yourself wide awake in the middle of the night, feeling a bit miserable and unable to get back to sleep.

Sleep is not just a pillar of good health...

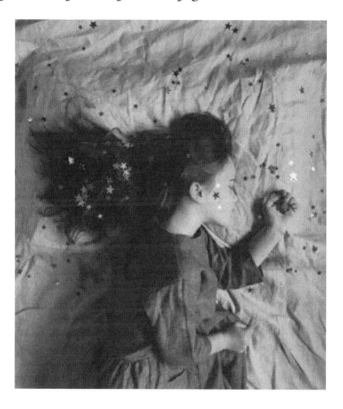

...it's the foundation

Stop the Vicious Cycle

It becomes a vicious cycle: the more you put in your bucket, the more time you spend in the negative primitive part of your mind, the more you're encouraged to think negatively...

Our thoughts determine our feelings and drive our actions

So it's time to be more conscious of your thoughts, to learn to choose your thoughts with awareness of their power - because the concepts and beliefs you accept with feeling inevitably become your own living reality. How you choose to think today influences all your tomorrows.

When you focus on your problems, you drag them into the future with you and they attract more of the same - your own thought patterns provide the energy that feeds your problems and keeps them alive.

By switching the polarity around, by consciously operating from the intellectual part of the brain, making positive, logical decisions rather than emotional, reactive ones, you start to focus on how you want things to be rather than on how you don't want them to be - and you start to attract the solutions.

By being more aware of your thoughts and feelings, you gain control instead of being controlled.

On a physiological front, changing the hormones that are released has a profound effect on how well you cope in life. By remaining in a stressed-out position, you will be releasing cortisol which keeps those feelings of threat, negative thinking and emotional reactivity at the fore. To counter-balance the release of cortisol you can work on releasing the most important neurotransmitter we have - serotonin.

When we have a constant supply of serotonin, we are happier, better able to cope and feel braver, it's our go-to hormone to keep us on an even keel and it acts as a catalyst for mentally healthy behaviour.

Just as we release cortisol when we're stressed, in order to get us ready for action, as you might expect serotonin is released when we're relaxed, when we're operating from the intellectual part of the brain rather than the emotional survival part.

When we practise...

- **Positive Interaction**
- **Positive Activity**
- **Positive Thinking**

... we produce patterns in the brain that give that constant flow of serotonin. Having that flow helps to cap the release of cortisol - when we don't have any serotonin in our system, cortisol can go on being released unchecked which ramps up the stress and locks you in that vicious cycle of negativity.

Finally, if we are relaxed we cannot be stressed, they are mutually exclusive states. Learning how to relax is therefore a crucial first step in overcoming stress - once calm, you can deal with the source of the stress.

CHAPTER 4:
SIGNS & SYMPTOMS OF STRESS OVERLOAD

The bio-chemicals that help us to cope with rapid change are:

Adrenaline – alerts us, readies us for action, increases our heart rate and blood pressure and mobilises our energy reserves

Cortisol – replenishes energy supplies and alerts the immune system to possible bacterial or viral attack or injury

When a stressful situation is resolved through action, the body and mind re-balances itself to homeostasis and no harm is done.

However if the perceived danger is prolonged or action is impossible, the hormones continue to circulate (for around 2 hours) and repeated release of cortisol causes the symptoms of chronic stress. This can result in impaired physical health as the stress hormones damage the immune system, making us vulnerable to infection, disease (inflammation linked with heart disease), and chronic pain (often back pain, fibromyalgia or migraine headaches).

As well as physical issues, prolonged stress can lead to depression and problems with addictions or compulsive disorders as we try to find other ways out of our stressful situation. Many addictions (such as alcohol, nicotine, drugs or food), often lead on to physical illness as well.

A key point in spotting stress overload or mental health issues in others is noticing any changes in behaviour or appearance that are out of the ordinary or without any obvious explanations. It is very hard to self-diagnose when you're in the middle of feeling overloaded because we tend to move into a blinkered outlook, keeping our heads down and trying to get by. It may be that the first time you notice stress overload in yourself is when someone remarks that you're not your usual self.

Everyone is different and reacts in their own way to stress, this is a list of common signs* and symptoms** but it's not exhaustive:

Emotional
Low mood
Feelings of irritability
Edginess
Anxiety or hostility
Over-alertness
Jumpiness
Feeling nervous, fearful or cynical
Lacking your usual sense of humour and sense of self
Lacking a sense of direction
Feeling unmotivated
Feeling depressed

*signs are things that other people can see (i.e. flushed face)
**symptoms are things that we feel but may not be detected by others (i.e. pounding heart)

Physical

Pounding, rapid or uneven heartbeat

Sweaty palms, sweating

Dilated pupils

Shortness of breath

Fast, shallow breathing

Tense, painful muscles

Tightness in chest

Muscle weakness, trembling

Headaches

Nausea

Skin rashes

Cold hands

Weakness in limbs

Tingling, pins and needles

Aches, pains especially backache

Twitches or tics

Sleeplessness or oversleeping

Fatigue

Tiredness, weakness

Changes in appetite (over- or under-eating)

Worsening of existing conditions, pain or discomfort

Dry mouth or throat

Indigestion

Feeling sick

'Butterflies' in stomach

Upset stomach

Frequent urge to urinate

Constipation or diarrhoea

Behavioural

Forgetting to do stuff, losing concentration or perspective

Having difficulty thinking clearly or making decisions

Being disorganised

Snapping or losing your temper

Fidgeting or restlessness (over normal behaviour)

Being unable to see other points of view in a discussion

Habitually indulging in negative self-talk

Finding it harder than normal to do logical tasks

Relying on an addiction in order to 'switch off' or 'clear my head' or

'escape'

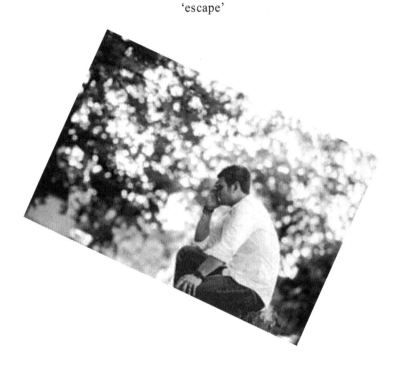

Setting your personal stress benchmark

Are there any gaps that you would like to work on? Remember that when we interact with others, when we're active and when we think in a positive way we released a flow of serotonin, the happiness hormone that keeps us on an even keel, better able to cope with life and it stops us remaining in the negative cycle.

Your Personal Stress Benchmark

	Low	High
Your thoughts - how positive have your thoughts been?	☐———————————————————☐	
Interaction - how interactive have you been with others?	☐———————————————————☐	
Activity - how would you rate your level of activity?	☐———————————————————☐	
Confidence - how would you rate your confidence?	☐———————————————————☐	
Strengths - how well are you utilising your strengths?	☐———————————————————☐	
Achievement - how much have you achieved?	☐———————————————————☐	
Happiness - how would you rate your level of happiness?	☐———————————————————☐	

Put an 'x' where you think you are on each scales

CHAPTER 5:
MEETING YOUR CORE EMOTIONAL NEEDS

We all have core emotional needs, and getting everyone's needs met is the basis for a healthy culture whether it's in the workplace, at home, or in a social setting. We might not consciously think about them being present but if they are missing we feel them through increased stress.

Our emotional needs are not hierarchical, they overlap and interconnect, but we need all of them to be met in balance to keep us well. If some of these needs are not met we can suffer emotional arousal which affects our rational, logical intelligence to drop, we become anxious, frustrated, distressed and angry which, if it's prolonged and not resolved, can lead to exhaustion, depression or various disturbing psychological states i.e. anxiety disorders, OCD, addictions, even psychotic breakdown.

Security - we all need a safe space and environment that allows us to live without undue fear, to develop fully and have space to grow. When we don't feel safe we fall back into our primitive brain, negativity dominates our thinking and behaviour, we are more likely to be fearful and aggressive or anxious and stress, and we are less able to make rational decisions. It occurs wherever security and safety is compromised, whether it's within families, at work or school or within our communities.

Autonomy - we all need a sense of control over what happens to us and within our environment, the freedom to make our own decisions and choices which helps us to feel in charge of ourselves rather than being overwhelmed by life, left helpless and frustrated that we cannot act on our own volition.

Attention - both giving and receiving attention are vital parts of our development. As new born babies we automatically seek attention in order to survive, and paying attention to each other forms part of our group bond as a tribal species, it helps us to maintain a shared sense of reality.

Intimacy - we are hard-wired for collaboration, finding emotional connections with others through friendships and loving relationships. We all need at least one other person who accepts us for who we are, the good and the bad. This may be our partner, parent, siblings, wider family, friends, neighbours, colleagues.

Community - connections with other people outside our immediate family i.e. work, hobbies, social activities, geographical. We have evolved as group animals because our survival in harsh conditions depended on us being part of a collaborative tribe. As primitive people, together we were strong but alone we were weak and at risk of death through predation or starvation, so even though we are no longer facing those life-or-death conditions we are still mortally afraid of being outcast from our groups - we have an innate need to belong to a group of some sort.

Status - we need to be accepted, valued and respected within our communities, to have status whether it's at work, within our families or friendship groups. Being respected for who we are and what we can do, how useful we are, by at least some people alleviates our feelings of being in danger of being thrown out or left behind by our tribes.

Achievement and Competence - having a sense of our own abilities, skills, knowledge and competence, without which we may feel inadequate, lack confidence and develop low self-esteem. We may withdraw ourselves from our communities if we don't feel useful enough. Genuine confidence built through demonstration of our competence builds our resilience, flexibility and spare capacity to cope with any difficulties.

Privacy - we all need enough time to reflect, learn and consolidate our experiences. In this modern world where our lives are held up for scrutiny on social media, privacy is an increasingly scarce commodity and needs to be carefully handled so that our minds don't become overloaded with a chaos of information.

Meaning and Purpose - which comes from being stretched mentally or physically, having purpose in what we do, being helpful in our communities or being connected to ideas/beliefs greater than ourselves (being interested in the world at large and seeing the bigger picture)

Assessing your core emotional needs

Thinking about your own life, how does each of the needs work in your life? Do you have enough security but not enough attention? Maybe you've neglected your need for intimacy by distancing yourself from your loved ones in favour of higher status at work?

You can assess each need on a Goldie Locks scale: too little, too much, just right - put an 'x' where you think you are on each need.

Your Core Emotional Needs

	Too little	Just right	Too much
Security			
Autonomy			
Attention			
Intimacy			
Community			
Status			
Achievement & Competence			
Privacy			
Meaning & Purpose			

Are there any gaps in your life, do you need to address any areas to find better balance? You can take this scale as an overall overview of your life or split it out across different areas i.e. scoring your needs within work only, or your home life.

CHAPTER 6:
BUILDING RESILIENCE

Now you know how stress works and you're getting an idea of whether your personal benchmarks are, how can you turn things around? How can you make the stress responses system work for you?

Remember the **'Doing-Driven' mode**? The stressed position that we often fall into operating from, where you are on auto-pilot, keeping your head down and getting on with it but not really being aware, not really enjoying life:

- Habitually responsive/reactive
- Over-analysing
- Continually striving
- Seeing thoughts and feelings as solid and 'real'
- Aversion to difficulty
- Mental time travel (past/future, not the now)

Firstly, it's not your fault…

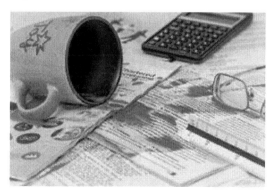

Life is really busy and really fast. Changes in the way we live have crept in, technology has ramped everything up we no longer shut the office door and leave work at the end of the day, we take it home with us, carried on our mobile phones or accessed from our tablets and laptops. And our home lives are busy too, with more entertainment at the tips of our fingers than our grandparents had in their lifetime, more opportunities to expand our knowledge, to look after our health and socialise.

But the number of hours in a day hasn't changed so something has to give. If you want to make sure it's not you, now is the time to address the situation, to assess whether you want to continue in that Doing-Driven mode or if you want to make a change, to emerge from the fog of busy-ness to being more aware, more present in your life - and less stressed.

Finding enjoyment again, getting back to the real you!

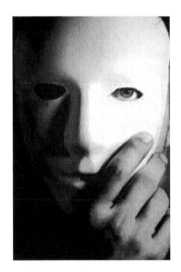

Changing to a more **'Thoughtful-Being' mode** where you are:

- Sensing, have awareness of yourself and your environment, your interactions with others (using your senses of taste, hearing, feeling, seeing, smelling)

- Accepting and being in the present moment (instead of panicking that you're going to be late, you have a more accepting attitude to things outside your control "oh dear, the lights turned red, never mind!", and you no longer do all that mental time-travelling which serves no purpose except to fill your stress bucket with useless worries)

- Approaching experiences with curiosity, rather than fear – this physically alters your hormonal balance (fear releases stress hormones like cortisol and adrenaline)

- Seeing thoughts and feelings as transitory mental or physical events, they're not solid or 'true' (they are your interpretation of events, not reality, and they don't last)

- You have conscious choice in our actions, based on a proper assessment of the situation using that logical, intellectual part of your brain

- Proactive as opposed to reactive, no longer falling back on emotional reactions that are not controlled by you but are a throw-back to our primitive ancestors' need to survive in a hostile world

Changing the way we think changes the way we act – because it changes the chemical balances we operate under.

CHAPTER 7:
MAKING CHANGES FOR A LIFETIME

This isn't about making sweeping changes in your life, upping sticks and moving to a deserted island, rather it's about changing your thinking and mindset about your life as it is, finding a new perspective so that you can make choices that work for you - instead of carrying on doing what you do just because you've always done it. Or if might involve making changes.

There are a wide range of tools and strategies you can use to take control of stress - again, this is not about removing all stress from your life, it's about learning to ride the waves of stress and build resilience so that you aren't broken by it.

Some will work for you, some won't, but if you keep an open mind and try them out you can make long-term changes in your life.

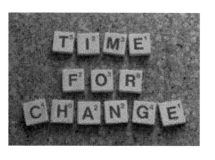

Accept it - Change it - Ditch it

If you are unhappy or feeling stressed whether it's at work or in your personal life, ask yourself whether you can accept the situation, change anything, or whether you have to ditch it altogether. These choices are not mutually exclusive - you might decide to accept a situation for now, knowing that something will happen later or you might try to change something but have to fall back on acceptance if it doesn't work out.

Be flexible - there is nothing so certain as change in our environment and a big part of our success as a species is our ability to be flexible and to adapt quickly. When things change we need to adapt accordingly if we want to not just survive but thrive - the flip side of this is that you might be frustrated at the lack of change or the slow pace of change.

- Accept what you cannot change, don't become easily irritated, don't set yourself up for chronic stress and possibly depression
- Be heard, give feedback if appropriate don't just grumble
- Check your facts, don't just assume
- Don't have untenable expectations, they lead to frustration, tension, anger
- Accept the imperfect world, tolerate ambiguity
- Remember, life isn't fair!
- See things from a different perspective, the bigger picture
- Maintain a positive attitude, nothing feels better when we're in a bad mood

Energy Management

We live in an era of constant interruption (continuous partial attention) from emails, telephone, texts, social media, apps, people...

Multitasking is a misunderstood term. We believe it to mean being able to deal with more than one task at a time, in fact we can only focus on one thing at a time but we can become adept at switching our focus quickly. However this is energy-sapping, leaving us ending our working day feeling exhausted and yet as if little has been achieved.

If you adopt one change, let it be this: **STOP MULTI TASKING!**

Assess your effort management: think about the value of each demand on your time and energy, ask whether it's really worth giving much attention to? Is it furthering your purpose or the purpose of the project or organisation?

Set time boundaries on electronic communication (metaphorically 'shut the door' on work) and use a buffer between work and home to separate the two - 20-30 minutes doing an activity you enjoy like exercise, listening to music, reading, whatever you enjoy doing that helps you to put work 'to bed' so that you can move into home life without any hangover (it works the other way too).

Listen to your rest-activity cycle

Our daily lives run on an ultradian rhythm: a recurrent period or cycle of approximately 90-120 minutes repeated throughout a 24 hour circadian day. During the night we have deep restful sleep interwoven with spikes of energetic REM dream sleep activity.

During the day the rhythm continues but with the onus on being alert most of the time, with energy dips every 90 minutes or so. The dips are there for a purpose, it's a time when our brains can process information received, integrate it into our innate map of reality, store useful stuff and let go of the rest, thus clearing our minds for the next active phase. It supports our night sleep, helping to process events and experiences out of the stress bucket so there is less to do at night.

In our modern busy world we can push through these dips, often using stimulants like caffeine and nicotine to do so but all stimulants work by stimulating the production of stress hormones, with all the attendant ongoing health issues. Quite apart from that, without these regular down times our spare capacity is reduced which will adversely affect our decision making, attention, temper, ability to build good relationships and overall perspective.

Whilst not suggesting that you take a pillow into work or take a nap during the day, allowing some time to break your focus, allow time for your brain to do a bit of free-wheeling will be hugely beneficial to your wellbeing and your productivity

"For often, when one is asleep, there is something in consciousness which declares that what then presents itself is but a dream."

– Aristotle, 322BC

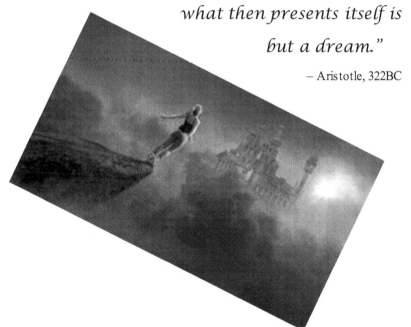

Ensure Lines of Communication are Open

Communication has been core to our survival, it's one of the reasons we have been so successful as a species. Allowing everyone to have their say and be listened to is a key skill in life both at work and in the home - effective communication avoids emotional arousal, criticism and contempt, and when done well can help to diffuse stressful situations.

- Avoid being defensive or stonewalling communication (blocking is a form of passive aggression)
- Don't ruminate, internalise or personalise
- Endeavour to have good relationships in all areas of your life
- Involve people, listen and remember to ask for help - people love to be helpful and being needed is one of our core needs
- It has a domino effect: one good relationship leads to another
- Remember that every human has the same needs
- And interacting with others, communicating with them, is one of the activities we need to do to create a flow of serotonin.

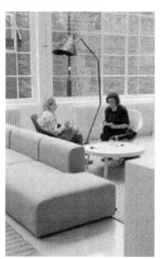

Avoid Work Stress spilling over into your Personal Life

How we see ourselves within our world is to a great extent influenced by our attributional style. This can be described in 3 P's:

Personal – how we react to adverse events or difficult situations depends upon how personally we take it. We can either think "it's all my fault, I'm a dreadful person" or "oh, that's unfortunate but I can see that it happened due to a variety of things"

Pervasive – our reaction also depends upon how all pervasive we think the adversity is. We can either think "this affects everything across the board of my life" or "this is unfortunate but here's a way around it and it doesn't affect the other parts of my life"

Permanent – our reaction also depends upon how permanent we think the adversity is. We can either think "that's it, my life as I had planned it is destroyed forever, or "that's sad but now perhaps I can move on and do something new"

Our attributional style can be altered through self-awareness and a desire to change. It is helped greatly if we are getting our emotional needs met in a variety of different ways, rather than just via one channel such as work.

Recognise our own Learned Conditioning, and that of others

We are all shaped by 3 elements:

- Our genetic inheritance
- Our interactions with our environment
- Our conditioning or learned behaviours

We cannot change our genes or alter what has happened to us in the past but

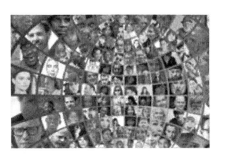

we can change how we perceive our past and any future interactions, and we can look at our conditioned behaviours with an open mind.

Becoming aware of our conditioning (our learned habits, beliefs and training through the circumstances of our upbringing) is a huge step forward in being able to change.

We all grow up in different circumstances and are shaped by different influences and with learned behaviours and habits - even siblings brought up in the same household will have different behaviours and views based on their own perceptions of their childhood. In essence we each create our own bubble of awareness that is unique to us - it's part of our stress footprint.

We each assume that 'our way' is best: learn to stand back and see the wider picture. It is possible to change your own conditioned responses and be more understanding of others.

Gain Perspective

When you're in the middle of a stressful situation, it's often very difficult to see the whole picture. Our stress response system is designed to spotlight the danger which is great when it's a predator standing in front of your but not so good when it's financial or relationship troubles.

Being able to stand back and gain perspective, to check the bigger picture, is a highly useful skill which needs to be developed under calm conditions and

practised regularly so that it can be utilised when it's most needed.

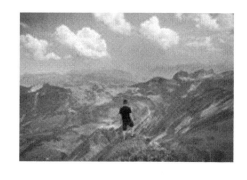

- Stand back from the situation with more detachment, to check the bigger picture. We call this our 'observing self' – a state where we are being aware and can look on at our own thought processes from an objective stance

- It's the opposite of being 'in flow' (totally absorbed in a task or event – which happens when you're in the auto-pilot mode)

- To have perspective you need to be working from the neocortex (intellectual brain), and not the primitive emotional brain

- To be a rounded human being it is vital to be able to enter both states at will: we need to be able to focus and get totally involved in doing things but we also need to be able to stand back and become aware of 'being'

Work Smarter not Harder

Whether at home or work, we all have schedules and timetables we need to operate around. Being effective in whatever you're doing is far more valuable than running around in a state of stress overload, it's the difference between being 'busy' and being effective.

- Plan your work don't let your work plan you
- Schedule your time
- Set yourself private periods in a hectic environment
- Learn to say 'no'
- Prioritise with the 4 D's of time management: Do it, Delegate it, Dump it, Defer it
- Don't let things build up and become overwhelming: Stephen Covey's Matrix of Importance vs. Urgency
- Set expectations and agree realistic deadlines, don't agree unrealistic ones
- Maintain a positive attitude, nothing feels better when we're in a bad mood

CHAPTER 8:
PUT YOUR OXYGEN MASK ON FIRST...
(before helping others)

Prioritising self-care can be tricky. It may bring up all sorts of feelings like guilt, and it can feel like you're trying to shoe-horn yet another activity into an already packed life - which only adds to the stress!

But while you're busy keeping those plates spinning and juggling all those responsibilities, and worrying that you can't stop for a moment otherwise it's all going to come crashing down, ask yourself this: what would happen if you fell over? What would happen if you suffered from serious mental or physical health breakdown? Who will pick everything up then?

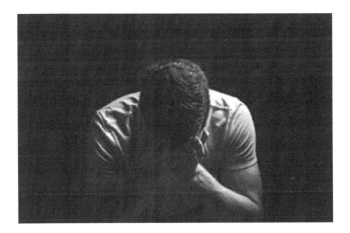

Self-care is not a dirty word, it is not being selfish or taking time away from your family or friends or work. Self-care is about making sure you are looking after your own health so that you can continue to care for others. And more than that, your family will appreciate you much more if you are well, full of vitality and happiness. This is about moving from 'coping' with life into 'thriving'.

So, before you even think about saying "I don't have time for this" consider how these things can be brought into your life in tiny steps ...

4 Pillars of Health

Nutrition, Exercise, Sleep, Relax - these are your 4 pillars of health. In order to be functioning well you need to take care of your greatest asset - you. Much the same as you'd make sure your car is serviced regularly, has the correct fuel, the brake pads and tires are changed, the MOT is up to date, so you also need to make sure your body is looked after.

Nutrition - we live in a sugar-saturated, convenience-driven world. It can feel like hard work to buy and cook from scratch but it really doesn't take that much time and can be used a part of your relaxation (I know, not everyone loves to cook but if you can change your mindset and embrace the activity instead of heading to the ready-meal section in the supermarket, you will feel the benefits!). Simple guidelines to follow:

- Eat a rainbow - include as many different coloured foods in your diet as you can, the more vibrant the colour the better (avoid large quantities of 'brown' or 'beige' food)
- Check the ingredients - try to buy foods with 5 ingredients or less, if you can't pronounce the ingredient you probably shouldn't be eating it
- Check the sugar content - low fat foods are notoriously high in sugar, try to stick to a ratio of 4g per 100g. A simple guide to reading the sugar content is to see how many grams of sugar minus any fibre to give you the amount of available sugar For example, a tomato has approximately 2.6g of sugar per 100g, less 1.2g fibre so the net sugar content is 1.4g of suger per 100g; Alpen Original has 23g sugar per 100g, and 7g fibre making net sugar 16g per 100g; Mr. Kipling cherry bakewell tart has 37.9g sugar per 100g and just 1.1g fibre, so the net sugar quantity is 36.8g per 100g.

- Drink before you eat - sorry, this isn't a beer, glass of wine or a G&T before dinner! Often when we feel pangs of hunger we're actually dehydrated so have a glass of water first.

- Reduce your plate size - we've become used to large portion sizes, reducing the size is an easy way of reducing calories without really noticing it. Remember: there's no difference in putting excess food in your waist (bin) and the waste bin! Over-eating becomes a habit that is hard to break

- Feed your brain - your brain cells are made up of water and approximately 60% fats, so you need good quality fats to maintain brain health. Foods like olive oil, avocado, coconut oil, and nuts and seeds (high in fats and minerals like zinc, copper, magnesium, iron), fatty fish (wild salmon, trout, sardines high in omega-3 fatty acids), colourful berries high in antioxidants like blueberries, spices like turmeric (antioxidant and anti-inflammatory), green leafy veg like cabbage and broccoli (fat-soluble vitamin K), dark chocolate, eggs, green tea - and caffeine

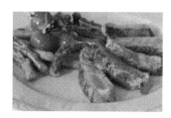

Exercise - positive activity is one of the ways we increase the flow of serotonin, our happy hormone.   This doesn't mean going to the gym for 3 hours 5 times a week, it means bringing movement into your life.   Whether it's taking the stairs instead of the lift or parking a little further away so you have to walk more, joining a dance class or doing yoga at home, moving your body every day is a good habit to get in to.   Start small and build on it, and think about activities that you used to enjoy but got forgotten by the wayside as your life changed - particularly good are group or team activities as you include positive interaction along with the activity but whatever works in your life.   And there are numerous home-based activities available online like 7-minute HiiT circuits, 20 or 30 minute yoga flows (or longer) - you can fit a bit of movement into your life.

Another motivator is to enter a race, whether its parkruns or local triathlons, cycle or running events, there are numerous events going on throughout the year. Having a deadline booked is a great motivator to get you going – or just get out and walk the dog.

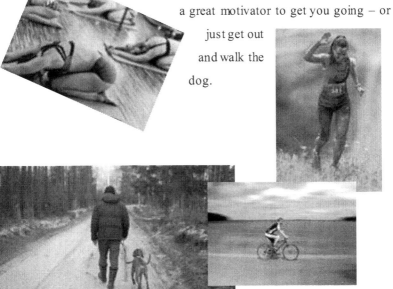

Sleep - this is arguably the <u>foundation</u> of good health, rather than just a pillar. Without proper sleep, we have a tendency to eat badly, falling back on high sugar foods to supplement flagging energy levels, we struggle to exercise as we don't feel much like doing it when we're too tired, and rather than relaxing, doing activities that help to calm the mind, we might simply end up falling asleep.

Sleep deprivation affects many **cognitive and physical functions**:

- **Memory Issues** – during sleep your brain forms connections that help you process and remember new information, a lack of sleep can negatively impact both short- and long-term memory
- **Trouble with Thinking and Concentration** – impacts concentration, creativity and problem-solving skills
- Mood Changes – become more moody, emotional and quick-tempered, which may escalate into anxiety or depression
- **Accidents** – being drowsy during the day can increase your risk of accidents and injuries
- **High Blood Pressure** – less than 5 hours of sleep per night increases risk of high blood pressure
- **Weakened Immunity** – weakens immune system's defence against viruses like those that cause the common cold or flu, you're more likely to get sick when exposed to those germs
- **Risk of Diabetes** – affects body's release of insulin, the blood sugar-lowering hormone. People who don't get enough sleep have higher blood sugar levels and an increased risk of type 2 diabetes
- **Weight Gain** – the chemicals that signal when you're full are off balance, as a result you're more likely to overindulge. You also tend to eat more to replenish flagging energy levels.

- **Low Sex Drive** – lower libido, in men this decreased sex drive may be due to a drop in testosterone levels
- **Risk of Heart Disease** – increased blood pressure and higher levels of chemicals linked to inflammation, both of which play roles in heart disease
- **Poor Balance** – affects balance and coordination, making you more prone to falls and other physical accidents

Since our primitive ancestors first harnessed the power of fire, we have been pushing back the night to augment the day. And in today's time-poor society we regularly steal from the night, staying up late to watch tv, socialising late, working and studying into the night... which impacts on the opportunity our brain has for that important stress bucket emptying as well as affecting the maintenance activities that happen overnight, such as removing toxin build-up and strengthening synapse connections.

Sleep hygiene tips:

- Prioritising sleep is a key element to maintaining good health both mentally and physically.
- Make your bedroom a 'boredom' zone, remove TV's/ipads, etc
- Keep your bedroom dark, use blackout blinds and remove any tech that has stand-by lights
- Keep your bedroom cool, optimum temperatures between 16-18oC

- Use an old fashioned alarm clock, not your phone - just having your phone by your bed whether it's off, in flight-mode or on, encourages the brain to seek it out. People who have their phone in their bedroom often look at it last thing at night and first thing in the morning, meaning you are forming a habit based on dependency rather than conscious choice

- Prepare your body by dimming the lights around an hour before it's time to sleep, this promotes the release of melatonin, the hormone that makes us sleepy. Blue light from digital devices, flickering tv screens and bright room lights all inhibit the release, tricking the body into thinking it is still daytime. You can also prepare by having a warm/hot bath (it's better to have a warm or hot bath or shower before bedtime as it tricks the body into thinking the ambient temperature is warmer than it is, it causes the body to cool down which is a precursor for falling asleep (our body temperature naturally drops when we sleep)

- Prepare your mind with soothing activities before bedtime. things like reading or gentle yoga, meditation, gratitude journaling, breathing techniques, body scanning, counting (backwards), or relaxation audios

Routine is key - just like you would have a bedtime routine for young children to prepare them for bed so we adults also benefit from routine, it prepares the brain for settling down into sleep.

Relaxation - this is probably the most misinterpreted and therefore the most ignored of the 4 pillars. Relaxation means different things to different people: ask a child how they relax and they'll probably say they jump on a trampoline or play football or run around the park; ask an adult and they'll say anything from reclining with a good book to watching a movie, practising yoga or going for a run. It's really about doing something that you enjoy doing, just for you.

In principle it doesn't involve digital tech (although that is truly hard to do given our music and entertainment choices are getting more digitalised). But it is about reconnecting with your real world and the people in it, rather than burying your head in a virtual life. One key element is that doing real life activities brings your attention to the now, and it is driven by your imagination.

Think about reading a book: as you read you imagine the story unfolding in your mind's eye, what the people look like, their environment, what they're doing. Your brain loves working out puzzles so it leaps ahead, makes assumptions, returns to the narrative. That's why we love twists and turns, surprises and also complete endings that tie everything neatly together - and why cliff hangers are so powerful, they keep your brain in a state of suspension, stuck at a crucial point in the story and desperate to know more!

Primarily when talking about digital tech, in this context it is directed at social media. With social media everything is being presented to you and you're being lead to the next offering, think about times when you've scrolled through posts - remember, social media is highly sophisticated, using algorithms that 'learn' your preferences so that it locks you into an information bubble that is unique to you. It keeps pushing more of what it thinks you want in front of you which means your brain doesn't get any puzzle to solve and you get pigeon-holed, more of the same kind of information is presented because that's what it 'thinks' you like.

We are also being conditioned by the imperative of the 'ping' - those new notifications and messages flashing to inform us that there's something we've got to see, right now! It's an updated version of an experiment that Russian physiologist, Ivan Pavlov, carried out with dogs during the 1890's - whenever he fed his dogs he used a metronome so that they associated food with the ticking sound it made. Eventually whenever he set the metronome, the dogs started salivating even without the physical food in front of them, they were conditioned by the sound to have a physical reaction, proving that a conditioned stimulus results in a conditioned response. And that's what happens with the ping of social media - we are conditioned by the sound to react (in our case it's a release of cortisol, the stress hormone), which gives us the urge to go check that phone!

Another reason people struggle with relaxation is they feel selfish - do something for me? I don't have time, I've got a million and one other things I've got to do to keep my life on track! But ask yourself this: what happens if you fall over with stress overload, who will keep things on track then? Spending just 15 minutes a day could make all the difference (let's start small here, you can build on it as you get used to the idea!).

The principle reason why you want to prioritise spending a short time relaxing is because it helps reduce cortisol by switching off an over-active stress response system. And, as with any repeated activity, the more you do it the easier it becomes to do, the more habituated your body and mind becomes to it. This is about creating new habits of behaviour that change your thought patterns that alter your chemical signature.

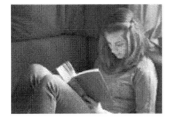

It changes your chemical responses, dampening down the stress response and its attendant release of cortisol and adrenaline, supporting instead the release of serotonin and a whole host of other 'feel good' chemicals'. It encourages you to remain more in the intellectual part of your brain (the logical, reasonable, positive part) and less in the emotional, negative primitive part of your brain. You are using neuro-plasticity to physically change your brain. And it impacts on your non-essential systems like the digestive system, the immune system, the reproductive system (all of which are 'switched off' when you're under stress), it supports your sleep, it re-sets your balance.

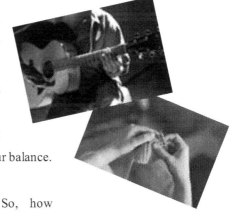

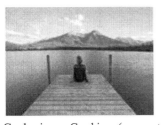

So, how will you choose to relax? Go for a walk - Play music - Sit down and have a coffee - Relax in the park in the sunshine - Read a magazine or book - Dance - Sing - Gardening - Cooking (see note in 'nutrition' about cooking as relaxation) - Meditation - Arts & Crafts - Knitting - Journaling - Breathing - Yoga - Tai chi - Holding a conversation with a loved one - Eat dinner every night at the table - Take the dog for a walk - Play with your cat - Learn a new skill...

Practise Positive interaction, Positive Activity, Positive Thinking

These three activities were introduced back under the explanation of our brilliant but imperfect brains - it's small steps we can introduce to stop over filling the stress bucket we all have.

Our primitive ancestors used these three activities to create positive patterns in the brain that promoted their wellbeing, helped them cope with day to day activities, it made them feel braver and it even helped them through physical pain - because these thought patterns cause the release of serotonin, the happy hormone.

So make sure each day has an element of **positive interaction** - if you work from home, use local cafes occasionally, use manned check-out tills rather than self-service at supermarkets, walk your dog where you'll meet other dog walkers, join exercise classes, and if you work in an office, take time to interact with your colleagues, ask them about their weekends, about their interests and hobbies as well as talking about work. Make sure you get your fix of positive interaction every day.

Incorporate **positive movement** into your life, as mentioned before this doesn't have to be long sessions in a gym, just bring movement into your daily habits - and think of it as movement rather than exercise, you'll find it a lot easier to fit in throughout your day.

Think about three positive things at the end of each day, acknowledge it. These are not firework moments but little things that gave you a small amount of pleasure: when someone said thank you, when you smiled at a stranger in passing, if someone holds the door for you or lets you into traffic, a colleague or manager or client compliments you on your work, your partner says 'I love you', your child gives you a hug, the sun came out, the birds were tweeting... we can all find so many moments if we only notice them. And acknowledging them just before you go to sleep either just quietly to yourself in your mind or using a gratitude journal, whatever works for you, is a great way to go to sleep because your brain will process those thoughts, it will start to change it's focus from naturally negative to being more positive.

These things may sound woolly, but they are rooted in science and have a profound effect on your physiology, through the changes in thought patterns and in the hormones being released. Remember: you practise to be the person you become. When you start thinking and being more positive in your outlook, it becomes your habit.

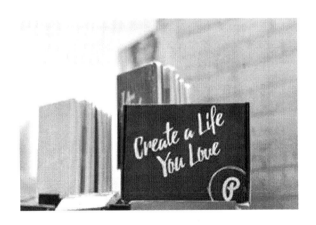

Nurture your relationships

Our lives are filled with relationships, from the moment you came into the world you have sought to build relationships with your close family, your very survival depended on it for your sustenance, warmth and shelter. As you pushed out into the world your connections grew, you aligned yourself with various friends and groups, even when you thought you were a rebel, beating your own path, you nonetheless identified with certain characteristics and group emblems (the make up or clothes you wore, how you styled your hair, the music you listened to).

We all have an innate fear of being left behind, of being thrown out of our tribes, vulnerable to death by predation or starvation. We are constantly seeking approval, to fit in, with our peers, checking who is stronger than us (who can protect us), and who is weaker (who makes us look better), all on an unconscious level. Our relationships matter to our mental health, as much as the food we eat and the air we breathe does to our physical health.

So it makes sense to nurture our relationships, to strengthen bonds with our close friends and family, to unite with our work colleagues, to be open to new connections.

- Don't be afraid to ask for help – from managers, friends, colleagues, family. Most problems feel better when it's shared, and you're giving them a valuable opportunity to be needed (something we all thrive on)
- Be yourself - people are drawn to authenticity and it is simply too exhausting to maintain a facade of someone you are not, it will slip eventually.

- If a friend or colleague acts out of character, don't take things personally, ask first before you assume. You don't always know what's been happening in their lives - they might need a hand of friendship rather than a cold shoulder.

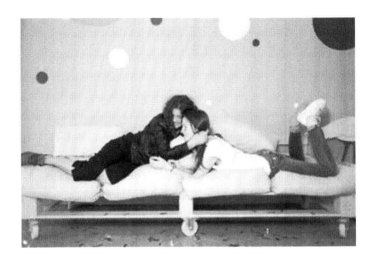

Feed your mind

Practices such as mindfulness and meditation are often misunderstood. They may be seen as 'woolly', hippy-dippy, new age spiritual beliefs that just don't work for you, but before you dismiss them out of hand, it would be wise to know what exactly they are.

Mindfulness is about being aware, being present, and can be practised both informally and formally;

- Formal practice: mindfulness meditation (see below under meditation)
- Informal practice: attempting to be more aware in everything that you do, throughout your day: eating, drinking, being with your friends or family, walking the dog, being at work, doing the washing up....

We do so many things in auto-pilot mode not paying attention to what is happening or what we're doing or experiencing. Mindfulness is an integrative, mind-body approach to life that helps people relate to experiences throughout the day. It means paying attention to your thoughts, feelings and body sensations in a way that can increase awareness.

Meditation, or rather Mindfulness Meditation, is probably most commonly thought of as 'classic' meditation (setting aside time to be still and focus on the act of meditating, bringing your complete attention to the present experience, clearing the mind) but actually, at its core, meditation is simply 'setting aside time to do something good for yourself', a bit like relaxation (see information for relaxation under the Chapter 8's 4 pillars of health).

For example:

exercise meditation (intentionally setting out to exercise, clear the mind, things like running that allows the brain to freewheel or weight training which is more focused, often based around counting reps)

- music meditation immersing yourself in music, particularly music that relaxes or provides a vibration such as om chanting, world music, Tibetan bowl music, etc - but whatever music you enjoy is good)

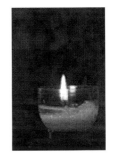

- prayer meditation (intentionally sending prayers out to the universe, probably thought of as 'classic' meditation)

We tend to think of meditation as a long process, taking a long time to 'master'.

"You can't stop the waves, but you can learn to surf"

- Jon Kabat-Zinn, professor emeritus of medicine and the creator of the Stress Reduction Clinic and the Center for Mindfulness in Medicine, Health Care and Society at the University of Massachusetts Medical School – and the man now considered the godfather of modern mindfulness.

The point is to learn to be present to the point that, when you feel yourself reacting in a certain way later on, you're so aware of the 'now' that you're able to take a step back, and literally change your knee-jerk reactions. It stops your mind from overthinking, something we are predisposed to do which creates stress and anxiety all on its own.

Effectively it teaches you to recognise the thought and change your reaction.

For example, you might habitually think: "I'm on a deadline, I might lose my job if I don't get it done in time, and it will be a disaster!" which activates the stress system (fight/flight response), stress hormones start flowing, you notice sweaty palms, a raised heart rate, churning stomach and you become more anxious which affects your ability to focus and be productive, and more negative thoughts intrude.

Instead you think: "Oh, there's that thought, blowing things out of proportion again, but it's just that, a thought, and not reality." which prompts you to step back and take a breath, regroup and refocus, and your stress system stands down. It might mean you continue to do the piece of work, bring in help or flag up that it's not going to make deadline, whatever the best course of action is – but you can make a considered decision rather than spiral down into anxiety.

In essence you can change the way your brain works which may have great implications in particularly stressful times: meditation and mindfulness lowers the stress hormone cortisol, helps us sleep better, and rewires the brain with a host of positive emotional qualities. It physically re-shapes the brain (neuroplasticity), causing us to rely less on the flight/fight response part of the brain, and more on the intellectual, reasoning part of the brain… because when we are relaxed we are in control and better able to make considered decisions.

You can practise both mindfulness and meditation in tiny snippets throughout your day, you don't have to set great swaths of time aside:

- Every time the traffic lights go red, focus on your breathing, be aware of your body
- When you go to make a cup of tea, use the time it takes for the kettle to boil to close you eyes and do a body scan or breathing exercise or simply practise the art of stillness
- When you walk your dog instead of allowing your thoughts to tumble to the next chore or email you have to send, look around you, notice the trees, the path, the sounds, watch what your dog is doing, be in the present not the future or past
- When your partner or children come home, ask them how their day was and listen to their answer - instead of allowing your brain to skip ahead to plan dinner or think about unloading the dishwasher
- On the train or in the car, play your favourite music and really listen to the words, the sounds, immerse yourself in it
- Spend a couple of minutes just before going to sleep focusing on your breathing

There are moments throughout the day you can use, and you can create habits to introduce them. After all, you make a habit of brushing your teeth for 2 minutes twice a day - why not make a habit of spending 2 minutes on your mental health?

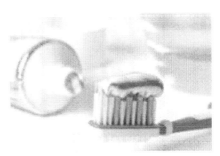

Your Life Support Structure

You may have already completed the two exercises earlier in this book - **Setting Your Personal Stress Benchmark** and **Assessing Your Core Emotional Needs** - if you haven't, it's worth going back and doing them. They will help you identify where you are now which is the first step to moving forwards.

Another area to look at is your support structure - **the Life House** is a valuable tool to assess where you might have gaps in your life, any areas you might want to work on to find balance. The more 'rooms' you have the more support you have available is, and the more stable you are likely to feel even if one room shrinks or disappears altogether.

Each room represents an aspect of your life - if all your needs are met through only one or two rooms (say work and family), then any trouble at work is going to leave you feeling vulnerable or unable to cope (think of the lights dimming in that room or turning off altogether, so you are reliant on just one area). However if you also belong to one or two clubs or have an active interest in helping others in some way, or are involved in the community, then your house will still be bright, the lights will be burning in those other rooms, making you feel more supported and less at risk of being overwhelmed by stress.

You also have more opportunity to focus attention away from the troublesome area, meaning you tend not to over-think things, you have a much better chance of bouncing back because your stress bucket doesn't get filled with useless worries.

These tools feed into your personal stress footprint, linking back to any gaps in your core emotional needs and your support structure... and you can review your personal stress benchmark, repeating the exercise to see where you are over a period of time.

So, now you can plan your future steps.

MAKING ROOMS IN YOUR LIFE

This is a Life House. Each of its rooms represents one aspect of your life.

A life house is a great way to visualise how you divide up your time. Each room in the life house lights up when there's activity occurring in it and each element, or person makes that room brighter.

If all your needs are being met through only a couple of rooms, then trouble in one will leave you feeling wobbly or anxious in the other. That's when you might feel the pinch of low mood swings, anxiety or depression.

Including clubs, engaging in active interests, community work or focusing on other aspects in your life increases the number of rooms in your house and makes the house brighter - even when one of the rooms has no lights on at all.

You also have a secret cellar. This is for anything you know about yourself that nobody else knows. It's important to acknowledge your secret cellar from time to time and re-evaluate what you keep here.

The next is 'me time' - reminders from the outside world. Reading, sports, music or meditation... whatever you enjoy.

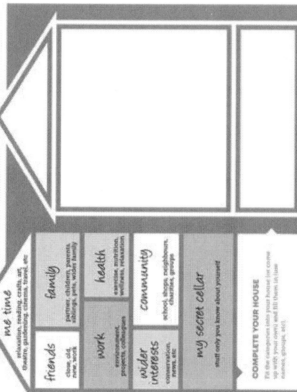

me time — relaxation, reading, crafts, art, theatre, gardening, cinema, travel, etc

family — partner, children, parents, siblings, pets, wider family

friends — close, old, new, work

work — environment, projects, colleagues

health — exercise, nutrition, wellness, relaxation

wider interests — conservation, news, etc

community — school, shops, neighbours, charities, groups

my secret cellar — stuff only you know about yourself

COMPLETE YOUR HOUSE — Fit the categories into your house (or come up with your own) and fill them in base rooms, groups, etc).

Geraldine Joaquim DSFH HPD

CHAPTER 9:
RECOGNISING YOUR FOOTPRINT

Let's start with whether you recognise the difference between operating from the intellectual, rational part of your brain and the primitive, emotional, fight-flight part.

Operating from a Driven-Doing Mode...
(refresh yourself by looking back at Chapter 2)

1)   Think about an event or experience you have had in the past when you had a strong emotional reaction. For example, a time when you were late for an interview or important meeting, or maybe it was standing up to give a speech, or you had an important project to manage.

Write it here...

2)   Revisit the scene in your mind, using as many senses as you can to reconstruct how you experienced the scene, try to remember the physiological signals you experienced at the time. This is your unique signature for that scenario and it's underlying feeling or emotion. For example, you may have noticed your heart beating fast, your hands were trembling, you needed the loo... you can look back at **Chapter4: Signs & Symptoms of Stress** but remember that is not exhaustive, you might have noticed other symptoms.

Write it here...

3)   Try to name the emotion. For example, you might have felt guilty for being late, or you wanted to avoid rejection, maybe you were anxious to do well or being competitive...

Awed	Belonging	Dislike	Inferior
Angry	Loving	Jealous	Afraid
Intimate	Competitive	Anxious	Shy
Superior	Affectionate	Guilty	Sad
Attracted	Rejected	Other	

...to a more **Mindful-Being Mode**

(operating from the intellectual brain - refer back to page 58 if you need to refresh yourself on what this is)

4) Having identified your emotion or feeling, note which of the following needs activated that feeling (refer back to Chapter 5: Your Core Emotional Needs for more detailed information on each):

Security	Privacy	Community connection
Autonomy	Attention (giving/receiving)	Competence/achievement
Status	Emotional intimacy	Meaning/Purpose

5) Take a step back from the named need, observe it in yourself and put it to one side

6)   Now that you have engaged with the scenario, identified your emotions and the need behind it, look back at the scenario and see if you could have handled it differently. For example, if you were running late for an interview instead of letting your anxiety run riot perhaps you could have thought about ways to alleviate those feelings, like calling the company to explain what's happened, or simply accepting that you can't change things outside your control.

Write it here...

What are your key stressors?

Identify what triggers you into stress - is it being late or being kept waiting, is it feeling like you have no control, is it relationships in the office or at home?

List everything you can think of.

-
-
-
-
-
-
-
-

How could you change the picture?

With each of the stressors, note down what would help alleviate them - if running late is your biggest stress, can you prepare earlier? If a relationship is at issue, can you approach the person involved? You don't have to actually do these things, this exercise is about being aware of possibilities - about changing your perspective.

-
-

-
-
-
-
-

Take a small step

Now think about one small step you could take to start you moving forwards. It can be related to the above stressors and solutions or something completely out of left-field - like cleaning out the kitchen cupboards. The point is to identify a small actionable step that you can achieve easily and quickly - because one positive step leads to another.

-
-
-
-
-
-
-
-
-
-
-

CHAPTER 10:
THE WAY FORWARD

Change is not easy and it's not necessarily quick, although it does often have a ripple effect. You will find that when you make a small positive change in one area of your life, it becomes easier to make others.

Think of it like climbing Mount Everest: no one leaps from the bottom to the top in one giant bound. They head for Base camp 1 first, settle there for a rest, then move to Base camp 2, rest, and on to the next one. Sometimes, if the going gets really tough, they might go back a step but they only go down to their last base camp, never right the way back to the bottom.

And sometimes they might not move directly from one base camp to the next, they might meander round the mountain, but they eventually move upwards until they reach the summit - that's where you'll find the real you!

And this analogy can be applied to making any changes in your life. If you shoe-horn in a big change it is unlikely the change will stick, you may see the positive effects for a short while but soon old habits bubble to the surface and are reinstated. Think of the many people who lose an amount of weight through a severe diet, only to pile it all back on and more... the change is not sustainable.

If you bring in small changes in steps, take time to consolidate them before moving forward to the next small step, you are much more likely to make long-lasting change. It is a gentler approach that uses your innate resources and systems instead of pushing against them.

Climbing Everest takes time, but if you do it well you will reap rewards that last a lifetime!

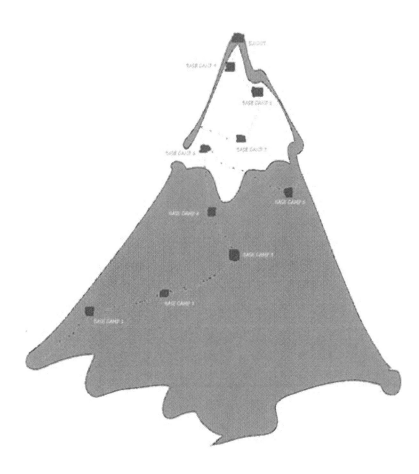

Be consistent

Recognising your triggers and being aware of the bigger picture is one half of understanding your stress footprint. The other half is understanding what keeps you well - looking after your health, nurturing your relationships, spending time on doing the things that make you happy - because those are the strategies and techniques that will keep you operating from your intellectual brain, rather than relying on the primitive, emotional brain.

And above all, make sure you **empty your stress bucket** (and prevent it from filling up with unnecessary negative thinking), and **keep practising Positive Interaction, Positive Activity and Positive Thinking** because these were the things that helped our ancestors thrive, they create patterns in the brain that promote positive mental behaviour - neuroplasticity at its best!

CHAPTER 11:
YOUR STEP-BY-STEP PLAN

7 Days to start climbing your mountain

Now it's your turn to start your mountain climb, changing your habits and moving you from where you are now to where you want to be. A calmer, more relaxed you – the real you who perhaps got lost along the way, through stress, routine, habits that you haven't necessarily consciously developed but nonetheless they shape your life. It's time to break free from those old behaviours that no longer serve you, and to instead consider how you want to be rather than how you don't want to be – or indeed, think about who you want to be rather than being the person you happen to be.

Spend 2 minutes every morning on this exercise:
First thing in the morning, ask yourself these questions:
What small step could I take to make a difference today, that would make we feel better, give me a boost? What would I notice that I would be doing, how will I notice that I am feeling happier, more positive, more confident?

If you're struggling to find an answer, think about what your preferred future looks like - what can you see yourself doing, what would your situation be, your environment, who is with you - what would you like in your life instead of the stress you have now?

And if you're really struggling to find an answer, look back on what you've already achieved, your past successes, what is already in your life that you appreciate, what has helped you in the past? And think about times when the stress wasn't there, identify specific times, what was different about that time, how did you make that happen? Re-framing your situation is a useful tool to help you gain perspective - we often think everything is bad, there's no way out, but if we can turn the problem around we begin to see alternatives, we see choices we can make.

Spend 2 minutes every evening on this exercise:
Just before you go to sleep, think about 3 positive things that have happened today. They don't have to be firework moments, major changes, just simple things that you noticed: the smell of a hand soap, a smile from a stranger, a seat that came available on the train, someone saying 'thank you', feeling sunshine on your face - they can of course be big things too - praise for good work, winning a new client, whatever you think is a positive moment today.

If you can't find a moment from today, think about a moment from the past that makes you smile - a holiday moment, a hug, it doesn't matter how big or small. The key point is to start recognising the good stuff, acknowledging it and looking for more.

The next few pages are for you to write those things down over the next week, to start changing the way your mind works, moving it from seeking the negatives in life to attracting the positive – and this isn't a woo-woo exercise, it's using your brain's neuroplasticity to physically change.

"It's not the mountain we conquer but ourselves"

- Edmund Hillary

7 Days to start climbing your mountain – Day 1

Every morning

What small step could I take to make a difference today, that would make we feel better, give me a boost? What would I notice that I would be doing how will I notice that I am feeling happier, more positive, more confident?

Think about the physical activity-based changes you would be doing rather than feelings, things like "I'd be taking time in the shower, not rushing through my morning routine." or "I'd sort out my desk, get rid of anything old that is no longer relevant and putting the rest away, filing it."

Write it here...

Every evening

Think about 3 positive things that have happened today. Write them down here.

1)

2)

3)

7 Days to start climbing your mountain – Day 2

Every morning

What small step could I take to make a difference today, that would make we feel better, give me a boost? What would I notice that I would be doing how will I notice that I am feeling happier, more positive, more confident?

Remember it's about noticing physical activity-based changes, not feelings.

Write it here...

Every evening

Think about 3 positive things that have happened today. Write them down here.

1)

2)

3)

Every morning

What small step could I take to make a difference today, that would make we feel better, give me a boost? What would I notice that I would be doing, how will I notice that I am feeling happier, more positive, more confident?

Write it here...

Every evening

Think about 3 positive things that have happened today.

1)

2)

3)

7 Days to start climbing your mountain – Day 4

Every morning

What small step could I take to make a difference today, that would make we feel better, give me a boost? What would I notice that I would be doing, how will I notice that I am feeling happier, more positive, more confident?

Write it here...

Every evening

Think about 3 positive things that have happened today.

1)

2)

3)

Every morning

What small step could I take to make a difference today, that would make we feel better, give me a boost? What would I notice that I would be doing, how will I notice that I am feeling happier, more positive, more confident?

Write it here...

Every evening

Think about 3 positive things that have happened today.

1)

2)

3)

7 Days to start climbing your mountain – Day 6

Every morning

What small step could I take to make a difference today, that would make we feel better, give me a boost? What would I notice that I would be doing, how will I notice that I am feeling happier, more positive, more confident?

Write it here...

Every evening

Think about 3 positive things that have happened today.

1)

2)

3)

Every morning

What small step could I take to make a difference today, that would make we feel better, give me a boost? What would I notice that I would be doing, how will I notice that I am feeling happier, more positive, more confident?

Write it here...

Every evening

Think about 3 positive things that have happened today.

1)

2)

3)

Don't stop now!

CHAPTER 12:
OUTSIDE HELP

There are numerous apps and platforms available in the wellbeing arena - things like Headspace or Calm, or hypnotherapy and relaxation audio downloads or cds.

These all help you to find space in your day to re-balance, and relax you for the night. This book comes with a hypnosis download which is designed to lead you gently into sleep, specifically the REM phase (that stress bucket emptying, brain processing time). If you didn't get it with the book and would like a copy, contact **geraldine@mind-yourbusiness.co.uk** simply stating where you got the book (i.e. attended a workshop organised by xyz company) and we'll send you an audio link.

To use it, simply play it when it's time to go to sleep (just after completing the nightly exercise of finding three positive things from the day is great). It's a series of language patterns that will help you drop off, it's not meant to be an active listening time, in fact the less you hear the better!

It may take a little while to get used to the routine of falling asleep to it but keep going, eventually this becomes your routine and your brain will switch off because it knows what is to come.

Additionally, the download can be used in the day if you have a spare 25 minutes or so - simply find somewhere comfortable to sit (you don't have to be lying down, just make sure you head and back are supported), and play the audio.

You will go into an altered state of consciousness, not asleep, but it mimics the REM phase, again for useful bucket emptying.

If you've ever driven from A to B and not remembered the journey, that's the same state you will be in, a kind of relaxed alertness where you still react to traffic lights, stop if a cat runs across the road and take the turns you need to. You will come back to full consciousness at the end of the audio but if you're at all worried about nodding off completely, set an alarm for 30 minutes.

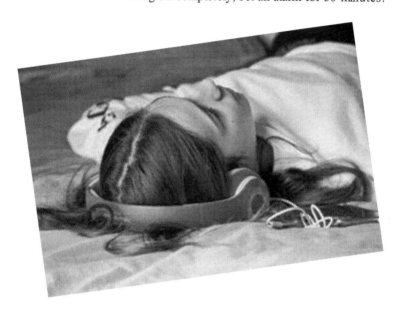

Needless to say, don't use the relaxation audio if you are driving or doing anything that requires your attention!

If you would like to seek more help to manage your stress, there are numerous therapies available. A good place to start looking is through the CNHC (Complementary & Natural Healthcare Council), an independent register of complementary healthcare practitioners which was set up by the government to protect the public. They set the standards that practitioners need to meet to get onto and then stay on the register, and all registrants are bound by the highest standards of conduct, are professionally trained and fully insured to practise.

https://www.cnhcregister.org.uk

There are also numerous associations around psychotherapy, I belong to the following:

- **Association for Solution Focused Hypnotherapy:**
  https://afsfh.com/find-a-therapist
- **National Council for Hypnotherapy**
  https://www.hypnotherapists.org.uk/
- **National Council of Psychotherapists**
  https://www.thencp.org/

I hope you've found the information in this book useful, and will explore what works for you to make changes to address your stress - remember there is no one-size-fits-all solution, it's important to find the strategies that work for you, in your own life.

Geraldine Joaquim DSFH HPD

Clinical Psychotherapist, Solution Focused Hypnotherapist and Stress Prevention Consultant

MCNHC MAfSFH MNCH MNCP

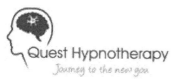

Quest Hypnotherapy Ltd
www.questhypnotherapy.co.uk
geraldine@questhypnotherapy.co.uk

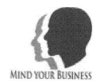

Mind Your Business
www.mind-yourbusiness.co.uk
geraldine@mind-yourbusiness.co.uk
(wholly owned by Quest Hypnotherapy Ltd)

Printed in Poland
by Amazon Fulfillment
Poland Sp. z o.o., Wrocław